Calisthenics For Strength And Mobility

A Complete Step-By-Step Gradual Workouts Guide For Strength Development At Every Fitness Stage

Vicky Klocko

Table of Contents

CHAPTER ONE

Introduction

Calisthenics is a form of exercise that utilizes your body weight for resistance training. It involves various movements and exercises aimed at improving strength, flexibility, and overall fitness. Instead of relying on weights or machines, calisthenics uses simple, yet effective, movements that challenge your body through different ranges of motion.

Principles of Calisthenics

Bodyweight Resistance: Exercises are performed using your body weight, making them accessible anywhere without the need for specialized equipment.

Functional Strength: Focuses on developing strength that's practical for daily activities, emphasizing movements that mimic real-life motions.

Versatility: Offers a wide range of exercises and progressions suitable for different fitness levels, from beginners to advanced practitioners.

Progressive Overload: Involves gradually increasing the difficulty of exercises to continue challenging your muscles and promoting growth.

Balance and Control: Emphasizes body control, balance, and coordination through movements that engage multiple muscle groups simultaneously.

Types of Exercises in Calisthenics

Static Exercises: Includes poses where you hold a position, like planks or static lunges.

Dynamic Exercises: Involves movements like push-ups, pull-ups, squats, and dips that utilize a range of motion.

Isometric Exercises: Focuses on contracting muscles without changing their length, such as wall sits or the "plank" position.

Benefits of Calisthenics

Improved Strength: Develops functional strength through bodyweight exercises.

Enhanced Flexibility: Incorporates movements that improve flexibility and range of motion.

Better Body Control: Enhances coordination, balance, and overall body control.

Minimal Equipment: Requires minimal to no equipment, making it accessible for all.

Calisthenics offers a versatile and effective way to improve overall fitness and strength while utilizing your body's natural movements. It's a great starting point for beginners and can be progressively advanced to suit individual fitness goals.

Methods/Styles used in Calisthenics

Street Workout: Incorporates freestyle movements using bars, benches, and other urban fixtures.

Gymnastics-Based: Involves movements inspired by gymnastics, including handstands, front levers, and planches.

Progressive Calisthenics: Emphasizes mastering foundational movements and gradually advancing to more complex exercises.

Each method/style has its own set of exercises and progressions, allowing individuals to find what suits their preferences and fitness goals.

Importance of Mobility

Enhanced Performance: Improved mobility allows for better movement execution and performance in calisthenics exercises.

Injury Prevention: Increased mobility reduces the risk of injuries by enabling a greater range of motion and better movement patterns.

Improved Technique: Better mobility helps in maintaining proper form during exercises, maximizing their effectiveness.

Functional Movement: Mobility exercises mimic real-life movements, making them essential for functional fitness.

Incorporating Flexibility Training

Stretching: Perform dynamic stretching before workouts and static stretching after to increase flexibility.

Yoga and Pilates: Both are excellent for enhancing flexibility and mobility through controlled movements and stretches.

Foam Rolling: Helps release tightness in muscles, enhancing flexibility and aiding recovery.

Dynamic Warm-Up Routines

Joint Mobility Exercises: Rotations and circles for shoulders, hips, wrists, and ankles to lubricate the joints.

Dynamic Stretches: Leg swings, arm circles, hip openers, and trunk rotations to prepare muscles for movement.

Movement-Specific Drills: Mimic the movements of the upcoming workout (e.g., leg raises, shoulder rolls) to activate relevant muscle groups.

A good warm-up routine gradually increases the heart rate, primes the muscles for action, and enhances blood flow, reducing the risk of injury during the workout. Combining dynamic warm-ups with mobility exercises helps achieve better flexibility and readiness for calisthenics routines.

CHAPTER TWO

Push-Up Variations and Progressions

Standard Push-Up: Begin in a plank position, hands shoulder-width apart, lower your body by bending elbows, then push back up.

Wide-Arm Push-Up: Similar to a standard push-up, but with hands placed wider than shoulder-width apart, emphasizing chest muscles.

Diamond Push-Up: Hands together in a diamond shape beneath your chest, targeting triceps and inner chest muscles.

Decline Push-Up: Feet elevated, hands on the ground, targeting upper chest and shoulders.

Progressions: Start with knee push-ups or incline push-ups if standard push-ups are challenging. Then gradually advance to the variations mentioned above, focusing on proper form and controlled movements.

Pull-Up and Dip Techniques

Pull-Up: Grip an overhead bar with palms facing away, arms shoulder-width apart. Pull yourself up until your chin clears the bar, then lower back down.

Use bands or assistance if needed to build strength.

Chin-Up: Similar to a pull-up but with palms facing towards you, emphasizing biceps.

Dips: Grip parallel bars with arms extended, slowly lower your body until elbows are at 90 degrees, then push back up. Use assistance or benches for support if needed.

Squats, Lunges, and Leg Strength

Squats: Stand with feet shoulder-width apart, lower your body by bending knees and hips, keeping your back straight, then return to standing position.

Lunges: Step forward with one leg, lower your body until both knees are at 90-degree angles, then push back up to the starting position.

Pistol Squats: Advanced single-leg squats where one leg is extended in front while squatting on the other leg.

Progressions: Start with bodyweight squats and lunges, focusing on form and depth. Gradually add resistance with weights or progress to more challenging variations like pistol squats or jumping lunges.

These exercises target major muscle groups, promoting overall strength and stability. Starting with proper form and gradually progressing in difficulty is key to mastering these fundamental exercises in calisthenics.

Muscle-Ups and Variations

Muscle-Up: Combines a pull-up with a transition to a dip. Start with a pull-up, then transition explosively to push your body above the bar.

Kipping Muscle-Up: Involves a swinging motion to generate momentum for the transition, requiring coordination and explosive power.

Progressions: Begin with mastering pull-ups and dips separately. Practice explosive pull-ups to chest height, then work on the transition between the pull-up and dip phases.

Handstand Progressions

Wall Handstand: Start with facing away from the wall, kick up into a handstand against it to develop balance and strength.

Freestanding Handstand: Once comfortable with the wall, practice freestanding handstands by balancing without support.

Progressions: Start with forearm or headstands for better control and gradually progress to handstands. Practice against a wall to develop confidence and stability.

Lever and Planche Training

Front Lever: Hang from a bar and slowly lift your body until it's parallel to the ground, engaging core and back muscles.

Back Lever: Hang from a bar and extend your body horizontally, facing the ground, engaging back and shoulder muscles.

Planche: Support your body horizontally above the ground on straight arms, engaging core and shoulder muscles.

Progressions: Develop prerequisite strength with exercises like tuck or advanced tuck front levers, skin the cat for back lever, and planche progressions like tuck planche or frog stand.

Tips for Advanced Training

Consistency: Practice regularly to build strength and skill progressively.

Proper Form: Focus on maintaining proper form to prevent injuries and maximize effectiveness.

Patience: Advanced moves take time and dedication. Don't rush; allow your body to adapt gradually.

Advanced calisthenics exercises demand significant strength, balance, and control. Progression through gradual stages and consistent practice are key to mastering these challenging movements.

CHAPTER THREE

Core Strengthening with Advanced Planks

Side Plank: Support your body sideways on one arm, keeping the body straight and engaging core muscles.

Plank Variations: Include plank rotations, plank with leg lifts, and plank with arm extensions to challenge core stability.

TRX or Stability Ball Planks: Utilize unstable surfaces or suspension systems to engage more stabilizing muscles.

Progressions: Gradually increase the duration or complexity of these plank variations to challenge core strength and stability.

Single-Leg Exercises and Stability Work

Single-Leg Deadlifts: Stand on one leg while hinging at the hips to lower the upper body, engaging hamstrings and glutes.

Pistol Squats: Advanced single-leg squats that require significant balance and strength.

Bulgarian Split Squats: Stand with one foot elevated behind on a bench or platform while performing a squat, emphasizing balance and stability.

Progressions: Begin with simpler variations and progress to more challenging exercises that emphasize single-leg stability and balance.

Enhancing Balance for Performance

Proprioception Exercises: Include exercises that challenge your body's awareness in space, like balancing on unstable surfaces (balance boards, bosu balls).

Yoga and Tai Chi: Practices that emphasize balance, coordination, and body awareness.

Dynamic Balance Drills: Incorporate movements that challenge balance, such as walking lunges, bear crawls, or one-legged hops.

Consistency and Focus: Practice these exercises regularly to improve proprioception and balance, which contribute significantly to overall performance in calisthenics.

Improving balance and stability involves training both the muscles and the nervous system to work together efficiently. Incorporating these exercises into your routine can significantly enhance your overall performance and reduce the risk of injury.

Common Injuries in Bodyweight Training

Shoulder Strains: Often due to improper form in exercises like pull-ups or handstands.

Wrist Injuries: Common in movements like push-ups or handstands, due to excessive strain on the wrists.

Lower Back Strains: Improper form during exercises like planks or back levers can strain the lower back.

Elbow Tendonitis: Overuse or improper technique in exercises like dips or muscle-ups can lead to elbow strain.

Recovery Techniques and Strategies

Rest and Recovery: Allow adequate time between workouts for muscles to repair and strengthen.

Proper Nutrition: Maintain a balanced diet to support muscle recovery and overall health.

Foam Rolling and Stretching: Aid in muscle recovery and reduce muscle soreness.

Ice and Heat Therapy: Alternating between ice and heat can help alleviate pain and reduce inflammation.

Pre-habilitation Exercises

Rotator Cuff Exercises: Strengthen the shoulder muscles to prevent injuries in movements like pull-ups or handstands.

Wrist Strengthening Exercises: Improve wrist flexibility and strength to prevent strains in exercises involving wrist movement.

Core Stabilization: Strengthen core muscles to prevent lower back injuries during exercises like planks or levers.

Injury Prevention Tips

Proper Form: Focus on correct technique to avoid undue stress on joints and muscles.

Gradual Progression: Avoid jumping into advanced exercises too quickly; progress gradually to allow your body to adapt.

Listen to Your Body: Pay attention to discomfort or pain; don't push through if something doesn't feel right.

Incorporating pre-habilitation exercises, prioritizing recovery strategies, and being mindful of proper form and gradual progression are key in preventing injuries and promoting overall well-being during bodyweight training.

Workouts for Busy Schedules

High-Intensity Interval Training (HIIT): Short, intense workouts incorporating calisthenics exercises like burpees, jumping jacks, and mountain climbers for efficient full-body workouts in a short time.

Circuit Training: Perform a series of calisthenics exercises back-to-back with minimal rest, targeting different muscle groups for a quick yet effective workout.

Tabata Workouts: Short bursts of intense exercises (20 seconds on, 10 seconds off) repeated for several rounds, allowing for a quick but intense workout.

Calisthenics for Travel and Outdoor Training

Park Workouts: Utilize playground equipment for pull-ups, dips, or step-ups.

Bodyweight Circuits: Create circuits using exercises like push-ups, lunges, squats, and planks that require minimal space and no equipment.

Resistance Bands: Carry portable resistance bands for added resistance during exercises like rows or assisted pull-ups.

Incorporating Bodyweight Exercises Anywhere

At Home: Designate a space for workouts; use chairs, walls, or the floor for exercises like squats, lunges, or wall sits.

Office Breaks: Incorporate mini-workouts during breaks, such as standing push-ups against a desk or chair dips.

Stair Workouts: Utilize stairs for step-ups, incline push-ups, or jumping exercises.

Tips for Consistency

Set Realistic Goals: Plan short and achievable workouts to maintain consistency.

Schedule Workouts: Allocate specific times for workouts to make them a priority.

Be Creative: Use your environment creatively to perform exercises anywhere and anytime.

Calisthenics' adaptability allows for workouts tailored to various schedules and environments. With a bit of creativity and commitment, it's easy to integrate bodyweight exercises into daily life, even with a hectic schedule or while on the go.

CHAPTER FOUR

Calisthenics for Specific Sports

Martial Arts: Calisthenics can enhance strength, agility, and flexibility important in martial arts like karate, taekwondo, or MMA.

Rock Climbing: Focuses on grip strength, upper body, and core, making calisthenics exercises like pull-ups and core strengthening beneficial.

Parkour and Free running: Requires agility, strength, and body control, aligning well with calisthenics' emphasis on functional movement and bodyweight exercises.

Combining Yoga and Calisthenics

Flexibility and Mobility: Yoga enhances flexibility and mobility, complementing calisthenics' focus on strength and control.

Breathe Control: Yoga's emphasis on breathwork can aid in better control and focus during calisthenics workouts.

Mind-Body Connection: Both practices encourage mindfulness and body awareness, enhancing overall performance and reducing the risk of injury.

Hybrid Training Methods

Weighted Calisthenics: Incorporating weighted vests, resistance bands, or ankle weights to add resistance and increase the challenge in bodyweight exercises.

CrossFit: Integrates calisthenics with other training modalities like weightlifting and cardio, providing a well-rounded fitness approach.

Functional Fitness: Blends calisthenics with functional movements to simulate real-life activities, emphasizing strength, flexibility, and coordination.

Benefits of Integration

Enhanced Performance: Tailoring calisthenics to specific sports can improve athletic performance by targeting sport-specific movements and muscle groups.

Holistic Fitness: Combining yoga and calisthenics fosters a holistic approach to fitness, balancing strength, flexibility, and mental focus.

Versatility: Hybrid methods offer diverse training options, allowing individuals to customize workouts based on their goals and preferences.

Integration of calisthenics with other training modalities can offer a well-rounded approach to fitness, catering to specific sport requirements or providing a holistic focus on overall well-being and performance.

Nutrition Tips for Bodyweight Training

Adequate Protein: Supports muscle repair and growth. Incorporate lean protein sources like chicken, fish, tofu, beans, and lentils.

Complex Carbohydrates: Provide sustained energy for workouts. Opt for whole grains, fruits, vegetables, and legumes.

Healthy Fats: Essential for overall health and energy. Include sources like avocados, nuts, seeds, and olive oil.

Hydration: Drink enough water to stay hydrated, as it's crucial for performance and recovery.

Timing: Consume a balanced meal with protein and carbs around workouts to fuel and replenish muscles.

Mental Preparation and Focus

Visualization: Visualize successful workouts, movements, and progress to enhance focus and motivation.

Goal Setting: Set specific, achievable goals to keep yourself motivated and focused on progress.

Mindfulness and Breathing: Practice mindfulness and deep breathing techniques to reduce stress and enhance focus during workouts.

Stress Management and Calisthenics

Exercise as Stress Relief: Calisthenics workouts can serve as a stress-relief outlet, releasing endorphins that improve mood and reduce stress.

Mind-Body Connection: Focus on the mind-body connection during workouts, using calisthenics as a form of active meditation.

Rest and Recovery: Prioritize adequate rest and recovery as part of stress management, allowing the body to recuperate.

Conclusion

Calisthenics isn't just about bodyweight exercises; it's a versatile approach to fitness that encompasses strength, flexibility, and control. From fundamental movements to advanced skills, its principles adapt to any lifestyle or fitness level.

Incorporating calisthenics isn't just a physical pursuit; it's a holistic journey. Nutrition, mental wellness, and consistency play pivotal roles alongside exercises. Whether you're striving for muscle gains, improved flexibility, or enhanced overall fitness, calisthenics offers a pathway toward these goals.

Remember, it's not just about mastering moves; it's about mastering your body.

The mental fortitude developed during training translates beyond fitness, fostering discipline and determination in all aspects of life.

So, embrace the versatility of calisthenics, integrate it into your routine creatively, and enjoy the journey of discovering the strength, agility, and balance your body is capable of achieving.

THE END

www.ingramcontent.com/pod-product-compliance
Lightning Source LLC
Chambersburg PA
CBHW061313250726
48653CB00002B/924